Snore-Free in 7 Days

Fast and Effective Techniques to End Snoring for Good

Solomon L. Bell

Table Of Content

COPYRIGHT ©   2

INTRODUCTION   5

UNDERSTANDING SNORING   5

CHAPTER 1   8

THE CAUSES OF SNORING: EXPLORING THE FACTORS THAT CONTRIBUTE TO SNORING   8

CHAPTER 2   11

THE RISKS OF SNORING: WHY IT'S IMPORTANT TO ADDRESS YOUR SNORING   11

CHAPTER 3   14

HOW TO DETERMINE YOUR SNORING TYPE: A GUIDE TO IDENTIFY YOUR SNORING PATTERN   14

CHAPTER 4   17

SLEEP APNEA: WHAT IT IS AND HOW IT RELATES TO SNORING   17

CHAPTER 5   20

LIFESTYLE CHANGES TO REDUCE SNORING: MAKING SIMPLE CHANGES TO YOUR DAILY ROUTINE   20

CHAPTER 6   **23**

BREATHING EXERCISES TO STOP SNORING: TECHNIQUES TO IMPROVE YOUR BREATHING   23

CHAPTER 7   **26**

USING ESSENTIAL OILS TO REDUCE SNORING: SAFE AND NATURAL REMEDIES TO HELP YOU SLEEP SOUNDLY   26

CHAPTER 8   **31**

ORAL DEVICES TO STOP SNORING: TYPES OF DEVICES AND HOW TO USE THEM   31

CHAPTER 9   **34**

SURGERY FOR SNORING: WHEN IT'S NECESSARY AND WHAT TO EXPECT   34

CHAPTER 10   **38**

HOW TO GET A GOOD NIGHT'S SLEEP: TIPS AND TRICKS FOR BETTER SLEEP   38

CHAPTER 11   **41**

CONCLUSION: YOUR 7-DAY PLAN FOR A SNORE-FREE LIFE   41

Introduction

Understanding Snoring

Snoring is a common issue that affects millions of people worldwide. It is the sound produced when air flows through the relaxed tissues in the throat during sleep, causing the tissues to vibrate. Snoring can range from mild to severe, and while it may seem harmless, it can have serious effects on your health and quality of life.

When we sleep, our muscles relax, including those in our throat and tongue. This relaxation can cause the airway to become narrower, making it more difficult for air to pass through. When air flows past these narrowed tissues, it causes them to vibrate, producing the sound we know as snoring.

There are various factors that can contribute to snoring, including age, weight, gender, nasal and sinus problems, alcohol consumption, smoking, and certain medications. In some cases, snoring may also be a sign of a more serious condition called sleep apnea, which causes repeated pauses in breathing during sleep.

Snoring can have several negative impacts on your health and well-being. It can disrupt your sleep and the sleep of your partner, causing daytime sleepiness, fatigue, and irritability. Snoring can also increase your risk of developing high blood pressure, heart disease, and stroke. It can even lead to depression and decreased quality of life.

But the good news is that snoring can be treated and even cured in many cases. With the right techniques and lifestyle changes, you can reduce or eliminate snoring for good, and improve your sleep and overall health.

In this book, we will explore various techniques and strategies to help you achieve a snore-free life. We will cover lifestyle changes, breathing exercises, essential oils, oral devices, surgery, and other solutions to help you stop snoring and improve your sleep quality. We will also discuss sleep apnea, its causes, and symptoms, and how it relates to snoring.

But before we dive into the solutions, it's important to understand your snoring type. There are different types of snorers, and understanding your snoring pattern can help you determine the most effective solution for you.

For example, if your snoring is caused by nasal congestion, using nasal strips or decongestants may help. On the other hand, if your snoring is caused by the relaxation of your throat muscles, tongue exercises or oral devices may be more effective.

In the next chapter, we will explore the causes of snoring in more detail and discuss the risk factors associated with snoring. We will also provide tips on how to determine your snoring type, and how to prepare yourself for a snore-free life.

So, are you ready to say goodbye to snoring and hello to better sleep? Let's get started!

Chapter 1

The Causes of Snoring: Exploring the Factors that Contribute to Snoring

As we discussed in the previous chapter, snoring occurs when air flows through the relaxed tissues in the throat, causing them to vibrate. This vibration produces the sound we know as snoring. But what causes these tissues to relax and narrow the airway in the first place?

One of the most common causes of snoring is excess weight or obesity. When we carry extra weight, it can put pressure on our airways, making it more difficult for air to flow freely. This pressure can cause the tissues in the throat to narrow and vibrate, producing snoring sounds.

Another common cause of snoring is alcohol consumption. Alcohol is a muscle relaxant, which means it can cause the muscles in our throat to relax more than usual, narrowing our airway and causing snoring. Smoking can also contribute to snoring, as it can cause inflammation and irritation in the throat, leading to narrowed airways.

Nasal and sinus problems, such as allergies or congestion, can also contribute to snoring. When our nasal passages are blocked or inflamed, it can make it harder for air to flow through them, forcing us to breathe through our mouths instead. Breathing through our mouths can cause the tissues in our throats to vibrate, leading to snoring.

Age is another factor that can contribute to snoring. As we age, our throat muscles become weaker and less toned, making them more likely to collapse and narrow our airways during sleep.

Finally, certain medications, such as sedatives or muscle relaxants, can cause the muscles in our throats to relax too much, leading to snoring.

It's important to note that these factors don't always work alone to cause snoring. Often, snoring can be caused by a combination of several factors. For example, someone who is overweight and drinks alcohol before bed may be more likely to snore than someone who only has one of these risk factors.

In addition to these common risk factors, there are several other factors that can contribute to snoring. For example, sleeping on your back can cause the tissues in your throat to relax and narrow your airway, leading to snoring. Sleeping with a pillow that's too high or too low can also contribute to snoring.

It's important to identify the factors that are contributing to your snoring, as this can help you determine the best course of action for treatment. In the next chapter, we will discuss the risks of snoring and why it's important to address your snoring. We will also provide tips on how to determine your snoring type, which can help you choose the most effective solution for your individual needs.

So, if you're tired of snoring and ready to take action, keep reading! In the next chapter, we'll dive deeper into the risks of snoring and why it's important to address them as soon as possible.

Chapter 2

The Risks of Snoring: Why It's Important to Address Your Snoring

While snoring may seem like a harmless annoyance, it can actually have serious consequences for your health. For example, snoring can be a sign of sleep apnea, a sleep disorder in which you're breathing repeatedly stops and starts throughout the night. Sleep apnea can lead to a range of health problems, including:

1. High blood pressure: When you stop breathing during sleep, your body's oxygen levels drop. This can cause your blood pressure to rise, putting you at risk for heart disease and stroke.

2. Diabetes: Sleep apnea has been linked to insulin resistance and glucose intolerance, which can increase your risk of developing type 2 diabetes.

3. Heart disease: Sleep apnea can cause changes in your blood vessels and heart rhythm, increasing your risk of heart attack, heart failure, and other cardiovascular problems.

4.   Depression and anxiety: The disruptions in your sleep caused by snoring and sleep apnea can lead to mood disorders like depression and anxiety.

5.   Cognitive problems: Sleep apnea has been linked to problems with attention, concentration, and memory, which can affect your performance at work or school.

In addition to these health risks, snoring can also affect your relationships and quality of life. Snoring can keep your partner awake at night, leading to resentment and relationship problems. It can also disrupt your own sleep, leaving you feeling tired and irritable during the day.

Given these risks, it's important to address your snoring as soon as possible. If you suspect you have sleep apnea, it's important to talk to your doctor about getting a diagnosis and treatment. This may involve undergoing a sleep study to monitor your breathing patterns during sleep.

Even if you don't have sleep apnea, there are still steps you can take to reduce your snoring and improve your sleep quality. In the next chapter, we will discuss the different types of snoring and how to determine your snoring type. This can help you choose the most effective treatment for your individual needs.

In the meantime, there are several lifestyles changes you can make to reduce your snoring and improve your sleep quality. For example, losing weight if you're overweight, avoiding alcohol and sedatives before bed, and sleeping on your side instead of your back can all help reduce snoring.

You can also try using devices like nasal strips, mouthpieces, and pillows designed to reduce snoring. These devices work by either opening your airways or changing the position of your jaw or tongue to reduce snoring vibrations.

In conclusion, while snoring may seem like a harmless annoyance, it can actually have serious consequences for your health and relationships. If you suspect you have sleep apnea, it's important to talk to your doctor about getting a diagnosis and treatment. Even if you don't have sleep apnea, there are still steps you can take to reduce your snoring and improve your sleep quality. In the next chapter, we will discuss the different types of snoring and how to determine your snoring type.

Chapter 3

How to Determine Your Snoring Type: A Guide to Identify Your Snoring Pattern

There are several different types of snoring, and understanding your snoring pattern can help you choose the most effective treatment for your individual needs. Here are some common snoring types and how to identify them:

1. Mouth snoring: Mouth snoring occurs when your mouth falls open during sleep, causing your tongue and throat tissues to vibrate. You can usually tell if you're a mouth snorer by the sound of your snoring - it tends to be louder and more open-mouthed than other types of snoring.

2.   Nasal snoring: Nasal snoring occurs when your nasal passages are partially blocked, causing you to breathe through your mouth instead. You can usually tell if you're a nasal snorer by the sound of your snoring - it tends to be quieter and more nasally than other types of snoring.

3.   Tongue snoring: Tongue snoring occurs when your tongue falls back into your throat during sleep, partially blocking your airway. You can usually tell if you're a tongue snorer by the sound of your snoring - it tends to be more guttural and throatier than other types of snoring.

4.   Positional snoring: Positional snoring occurs when your snoring is worse in certain sleep positions. For example, if you snore more when sleeping on your back, you may be a positional snorer. This type of snoring is often caused by the tongue falling back into the throat when sleeping on the back.

5.   Combination snoring: Combination snoring occurs when you snore in more than one way, such as both mouth and tongue snoring. This type of snoring can be more difficult to treat and may require a combination of treatments.

So, how do you determine your snoring type? One way is to record yourself sleeping and listen to the recording to identify the sound and pattern of your snoring. You can also ask your partner or a friend to listen and provide feedback.

Another option is to visit a sleep specialist or undergo a sleep study, which can monitor your breathing and help identify the cause of your snoring.

Once you've identified your snoring type, you can choose the most effective treatment for your individual needs. For example, if you're a mouth snorer, using a mouthpiece or chin strap to keep your mouth closed during sleep may help reduce snoring. If you're a nasal snorer, using nasal strips or a saline nasal spray to open up your nasal passages may be effective. If you're a tongue snorer, using a tongue stabilizing device or undergoing surgery to remove excess tissue may be necessary.

It's important to remember that snoring can have serious consequences for your health and relationships, so it's important to address your snoring as soon as possible. In addition to using treatments specific to your snoring type, there are also several lifestyle changes you can make to reduce snoring, such as losing weight if you're overweight, avoiding alcohol and sedatives before bed, and sleeping on your side instead of your back.

Chapter 4

Sleep Apnea: What It Is and How It Relates to Snoring

If you or a loved one has been diagnosed with sleep apnea, you may have heard that snoring is a common symptom. But what exactly is sleep apnea, and how does it relate to snoring?

Sleep apnea is a serious sleep disorder that occurs when a person's breathing is interrupted during sleep. This interruption can happen hundreds of times a night, and each time it occurs, it briefly wakes the person up, disrupting their sleep cycle. People with sleep apnea often don't realize they're waking up because it's such a brief interruption, but they may experience symptoms such as fatigue, headaches, and difficulty concentrating during the day.

So how does snoring fit into the picture? Snoring is often a symptom of sleep apnea. When a person has sleep apnea, the airway becomes blocked during sleep, causing a vibration of the tissues in the back of the throat. This vibration is what causes the snoring sound. However, not everyone who snores has sleep apnea and not everyone with sleep apnea snores.

There are two main types of sleep apnea: obstructive sleep apnea and central sleep apnea. Obstructive sleep apnea is the more common type and is caused by a blockage of the airway during sleep, usually due to the collapse of the soft tissues in the back of the throat. Central sleep apnea, on the other hand, is caused by a failure of the brain to signal the muscles to breathe during sleep.

If you suspect you or a loved one may have sleep apnea, it's important to speak with a healthcare professional. Diagnosis typically involves a sleep study, which can be done in a sleep lab or at home with a portable monitoring device. Treatment options for sleep apnea may include lifestyle changes, such as weight loss or quitting smoking, as well as the use of a continuous positive airway pressure (CPAP) machine, oral appliances, or surgery in more severe cases.

It's also important to note that untreated sleep apnea can have serious health consequences. It's been linked to high blood pressure, heart disease, stroke, and diabetes, among other conditions. Getting treatment for sleep apnea can not only improve your quality of life but also reduce your risk of these health problems.

In conclusion, while snoring can be a symptom of sleep apnea, not everyone who snores has sleep apnea, and not everyone with sleep apnea snores.

Sleep apnea is a serious sleep disorder that requires medical attention and can have serious health consequences if left untreated. If you or a loved one suspects they may have sleep apnea, it's important to speak with a healthcare professional and explore treatment options.

Chapter 5

Lifestyle Changes to Reduce Snoring: Making Simple Changes to Your Daily Routine

Many lifestyle factors can contribute to snoring, including being overweight, smoking, drinking alcohol, and sleeping on your back. By making simple changes to your daily routine, you can reduce your snoring and improve your overall health and well-being.

1. Lose weight: Being overweight can increase the amount of tissue in the throat, leading to snoring. Losing weight through a healthy diet and exercise can help reduce snoring and improve your overall health.

2. Exercise regularly: Regular exercise can improve your overall health and reduce snoring. Exercise can help you lose weight, tone your muscles, and improve your breathing.

3. Quit smoking: Smoking can irritate the tissues in the throat and cause inflammation, leading to snoring. Quitting smoking can improve your overall health and reduce snoring.

4.   Avoid alcohol and sedatives: Alcohol and sedatives can relax the muscles in the throat, leading to snoring. Avoiding these substances before bed can help reduce snoring and improve your sleep quality.

5.   Sleep on your side: Sleeping on your back can cause your tongue and soft palate to collapse to the back of your throat, leading to snoring. Sleeping on your side can help keep your airway open and reduce snoring.

6.   Elevate your head: Elevating your head while sleeping can help keep your airway open and reduce snoring. You can do this by using a wedge pillow or raising the head of your bed by a few inches.

7.   Keep your bedroom air moist: Dry air can irritate the tissues in your throat and contribute to snoring. Using a humidifier in your bedroom can help keep the air moist and reduce snoring.

By making these simple lifestyle changes, you can reduce your snoring and improve your overall health and well-being. However, it's important to remember that these changes may not be effective for everyone, and some people may require additional treatment to reduce their snoring.

Chapter 6

Breathing Exercises to Stop Snoring: Techniques to Improve Your Breathing

Breathing exercises can help improve the strength and tone of the muscles in your throat and reduce the likelihood of them collapsing during sleep, which is one of the main causes of snoring. Here are some breathing exercises that can help reduce snoring:

1. Tongue exercises: Stick your tongue out as far as you can and hold it for a few seconds before bringing it back in. Repeat this exercise a few times a day to help tone the muscles in your tongue and throat.

2. Lip exercises: Pucker your lips as if you were about to whistle and hold for a few seconds before relaxing. Repeat this exercise a few times a day to help tone the muscles in your lips and throat.

3. Breathing exercises: Take a deep breath in through your nose and exhale slowly through your mouth, making a "sss" sound. Repeat this exercise a few times a day to help improve your breathing and reduce snoring.

4.   Uvula exercises: Gently gargle with water while making a "k" sound to help tone the muscles in the back of your throat and reduce snoring.

5.   Yoga and meditation: Practicing yoga and meditation can help improve your breathing and reduce stress, which can contribute to snoring. Try incorporating some breathing techniques into your yoga or meditation practice to help reduce snoring.

It's important to note that while breathing exercises can be effective for reducing snoring, they may not be effective for everyone. If you have severe snoring or other sleep-related issues, it's important to speak with a medical professional to determine the best course of treatment for you.

In addition to breathing exercises, there are other techniques you can try to improve your breathing and reduce snoring, including:

1. Nasal strips: These adhesive strips are placed on the outside of your nose to help open up your nasal passages and improve your breathing.

2.   Neti pot: This is a small pot that is filled with saline solution and used to rinse out your nasal passages, helping to improve your breathing.

3.   CPAP machine: A continuous positive airway pressure (CPAP) machine is a device that delivers a constant stream of air pressure through a mask to keep your airway open during sleep.

4.   Oral appliances: These are devices that are worn in your mouth to help reposition your jaw and tongue to keep your airway open during sleep.

Breathing exercises can be a great way to help reduce snoring and improve your breathing. By incorporating these exercises into your daily routine and exploring other techniques, you can find the right combination of treatments to help you achieve a snore-free night's sleep.

Chapter 7

Using Essential Oils to Reduce Snoring: Safe and Natural Remedies to Help You Sleep Soundly

If you're looking for a safe and natural way to reduce your snoring, essential oils may be just what you need. These oils, which are extracted from plants, have been used for centuries for their medicinal properties. They can be used in a variety of ways, from diffusing them in a room to applying them topically on your skin or using them in a steam inhalation. In this chapter, we'll explore some of the most effective essential oils for reducing snoring and how to use them safely and effectively.

Peppermint Oil

Peppermint oil is one of the most versatile essential oils available, and it's an excellent choice for reducing snoring. Its anti-inflammatory and antispasmodic properties help to reduce swelling and relax the muscles in your nasal passages, which can help to reduce snoring. To use peppermint oil, you can add a few drops to a diffuser and inhale the scent before bed. Alternatively, you can mix a few drops with carrier oil, such as coconut oil, and apply it topically to your chest, neck, and temples.

Eucalyptus Oil

Eucalyptus oil is another essential oil that is excellent for reducing snoring. It's a natural decongestant, which means it can help to clear your nasal passages and make breathing easier. Eucalyptus oil also has anti-inflammatory properties, which can help to reduce swelling in your airways. You can use eucalyptus oil in a diffuser or mix it with carrier oil and apply it topically.

Lavender Oil

Lavender oil is well-known for its relaxing and calming properties. It can help to reduce anxiety and promote relaxation, which can make it easier to fall asleep and stay asleep. Lavender oil is also a natural anti-inflammatory, which means it can help to reduce swelling in your nasal passages and airways. To use lavender oil, you can add a few drops to a diffuser or mix it with a carrier oil and apply it topically to your chest and neck.

Tea Tree Oil

Tea tree oil is a powerful antiseptic and anti-inflammatory. It can help to reduce inflammation and clear your airways, which can help to reduce snoring. To use tea tree oil, you can add a few drops to a diffuser or mix it with carrier oil and apply it topically to your chest and neck.

Thyme Oil

Thyme oil is another essential oil that is excellent for reducing snoring. It has antispasmodic properties, which can help to relax the muscles in your throat and reduce snoring. Thyme oil is also a natural expectorant, which means it can help to clear mucus from your airways. To use thyme oil, you can add a few drops to a diffuser or mix it with a carrier oil and apply it topically to your chest and neck.

Safety Precautions

While essential oils are generally safe, it's important to use them properly to avoid any adverse reactions. Always dilute essential oils with a carrier oil before applying them topically, and never ingest essential oils. If you have sensitive skin or allergies, do a patch test before using any new essential oil. And always consult with a healthcare professional before using essential oils, especially if you're pregnant, nursing, or taking medication.

Conclusion

Essential oils can be a safe and natural remedy to reduce snoring. However, it is important to use them correctly and to test a small amount on your skin before using them on a larger area. If you have any concerns or underlying health conditions, it is important to speak to your healthcare provider before using essential oils.

Chapter 8

Oral Devices to Stop Snoring: Types of Devices and How to Use Them

If you've tried all the lifestyle changes and breathing exercises to reduce snoring and still can't seem to find relief, it may be time to consider oral devices. Oral devices, also known as mandibular advancement devices (MADs), are designed to help keep your airway open during sleep by holding your jaw and tongue forward. They can be an effective solution for mild to moderate snoring and may also be helpful for those with sleep apnea.

There are several types of oral devices available on the market, each with its own unique features and benefits. Here are some of the most common types of oral devices and how they work:

1. Mandibular Advancement Devices (MADs): These devices look like sports mouthguards and work by holding the lower jaw in a slightly forward position. This helps to keep the airway open and reduce snoring.

2. Tongue Retaining Devices (TRDs): TRDs are designed to hold your tongue forward to keep it from blocking your airway. They work by creating a

suction seal around your tongue and holding it in place.

3.   Palatal Implants: This is a minimally invasive procedure that involves inserting small implants into the soft palate. The implants help to stiffen the tissue and prevent it from vibrating during sleep, which can cause snoring.

4.   Continuous Positive Airway Pressure (CPAP) Machines: While not technically an oral device, CPAP machines are often used to treat sleep apnea, a condition in which the airway becomes completely blocked during sleep. CPAP machines work by delivering a constant stream of air through a mask to keep the airway open.

When choosing an oral device, it's important to consult with your dentist or sleep specialist to determine which device is best for your specific needs. They may recommend a custom-fitted device, which is designed to fit your mouth perfectly and provide maximum effectiveness.

Once you have your oral device, it's important to use it correctly to ensure optimal results. Here are some tips for using your device:

1. Follow the instructions provided by your dentist or sleep specialist.
2. Clean your device regularly to prevent bacteria buildup.
3. Practice wearing your device during the day to get used to the sensation before wearing it at night.
4. Start with a low level of advancement and gradually increase it over time.
5. If you experience any discomfort or pain while wearing your device, consult with your dentist or sleep specialist.

While oral devices can be effective in reducing snoring, they are not a cure-all solution. It's important to continue making lifestyle changes and practicing good sleep hygiene to ensure the best possible sleep quality.

In conclusion, oral devices can be an effective solution for those who suffer from snoring or mild to moderate sleep apnea. By working with your dentist or sleep specialist and using your device correctly, you can find relief from snoring and get the restful sleep you deserve.

Chapter 9

Surgery for Snoring: When It's Necessary and What to Expect

Snoring can be an annoying and sometimes even dangerous condition. If you've tried all the lifestyle changes, breathing exercises, and other non-invasive remedies without success, it may be time to consider surgery.

Surgery for snoring is generally reserved for severe cases where the snoring is caused by a physical issue that cannot be corrected with lifestyle changes or other non-invasive treatments. These issues may include:

- Enlarged tonsils or adenoids.
- Deviated septum.
- Narrow airway.
- Obstructive sleep apnea.

It's important to note that surgery is not always a guaranteed cure for snoring. However, it can significantly improve symptoms in some cases.

There are several different types of surgical procedures for snoring, and the type of surgery recommended will depend on the underlying cause of the snoring. Here are some of the most common surgical options:

1. **Uvulopalatopharyngoplasty (UPPP)**
   UPPP is one of the most common surgical procedures for snoring. It involves removing the excess tissue from the throat, including the uvula, tonsils, and part of the soft palate. This helps to open up the airway and reduce snoring.

2. **Radiofrequency ablation (RFA)**
   RFA is a minimally invasive procedure that uses heat to shrink the tissues in the throat that contribute to snoring. The procedure is done under local anesthesia and can be completed in a doctor's office.

3. **Palatal implants**
   Palatal implants involve inserting small rods into the soft palate to help stiffen it and reduce snoring. The rods are made of a biocompatible material and are usually well-tolerated by the body.

4. **Septoplasty**
   Septoplasty is a surgical procedure to correct a deviated septum, which can contribute to

snoring. During the procedure, the surgeon will straighten the nasal septum, which can help to open the airway and reduce snoring.

5. **Maxillofacial surgery**
   In some cases, snoring is caused by a structural issue in the jaw or face. Maxillofacial surgery can help to correct these issues, which can help to reduce snoring.

While surgery can be an effective treatment for snoring, it's important to understand that it comes with risks and potential complications. These can include bleeding, infection, and changes in voice or speech. Additionally, recovery times can vary depending on the type of surgery performed.

If you are considering surgery for snoring, it's important to talk to your doctor about the risks and benefits of each procedure. Your doctor can help you determine if surgery is the right option for you and can provide guidance on what to expect during and after the procedure.

In addition to surgical options, there are also several non-invasive treatments for snoring that may be effective for some people. These include continuous positive airway pressure (CPAP) machines, oral appliances, and positional therapy.

No matter what treatment option you choose, it's important to address your snoring, as it can have serious consequences on your health and quality of life. By working with your doctor and exploring different treatment options, you can find a solution that works for you and get the snore-free sleep you deserve.

Chapter 10

How to Get a Good Night's Sleep: Tips and Tricks for Better Sleep

We all know how important it is to get a good night's sleep. It's essential for our physical and mental well-being. However, if you're someone who snores or struggles to fall asleep, it can be a real challenge. In this chapter, we'll discuss some tips and tricks for better sleep that can help you overcome these challenges and wake up feeling refreshed.

One of the most important things you can do to improve your sleep is to establish a regular sleep schedule. This means going to bed and waking up at the same time every day, even on weekends. This helps regulate your body's internal clock, making it easier to fall asleep and wake up naturally.

Another tip is to create a relaxing bedtime routine. This might include reading a book, taking a warm bath, or practicing some deep breathing exercises. Whatever helps you relax and unwind, make it a regular part of your routine.

It's also important to create a sleep-conducive environment. This means making sure your bedroom is cool, dark, and quiet. Consider investing in some blackout curtains or a white noise machine if outside noises are keeping you up at night.

If you struggle with snoring or sleep apnea, using a special pillow designed to keep your airways open can be helpful. These pillows are designed to help you sleep in a position that reduces snoring and improves breathing.

Additionally, avoiding certain foods and beverages before bed can improve the quality of your sleep. Caffeine and alcohol can disrupt your sleep, so it's best to avoid them for several hours before bedtime.

Regular exercise is another great way to improve your sleep quality. Exercise not only helps you fall asleep faster, but also helps you stay asleep longer. Just be sure to avoid intense exercise close to bedtime, as it can have the opposite effect and make it harder to fall asleep.

If you're still struggling to get a good night's sleep, it may be worth talking to your doctor. They can evaluate you for sleep disorders such as sleep apnea and recommend treatments such as continuous positive airway pressure (CPAP) therapy.

In conclusion, getting a good night's sleep is essential for our overall health and well-being. By establishing a regular sleep schedule, creating a relaxing bedtime routine, creating a sleep-conducive environment, using special pillows, avoiding certain foods and beverages, exercising regularly, and seeking medical help, if necessary, we can all improve our sleep quality and wake up feeling refreshed and ready to tackle the day ahead.

Chapter 11

Conclusion: Your 7-Day Plan for a Snore-Free Life

Congratulations! You have reached the end of this book. By now, you should have a better understanding of what causes snoring, the risks associated with it, and various techniques to help reduce or eliminate snoring.

As a recap, we have explored the different types of snoring and their causes, from lifestyle factors to anatomical issues. We have discussed the importance of addressing snoring, not only for better sleep quality, but also to prevent potential health risks such as cardiovascular disease and stroke.

We have also discussed various ways to reduce snoring, including lifestyle changes, breathing exercises, essential oils, oral devices, and surgery. Each method has its benefits and potential drawbacks, but it is essential to find the right one that works for you.

Finally, we have touched upon sleep apnea, a severe sleep disorder that often goes hand in hand with snoring. If you suspect you may have sleep apnea, it is vital to seek medical attention.

Now, as promised, it's time to lay out your seven-day plan for a snore-free life. Here's what you can do:

Day 1: Determine your snoring type by using the techniques outlined in Chapter 4.

Day 2-3: Begin implementing lifestyle changes such as losing weight, avoiding alcohol before bed, and changing your sleep position (Chapter 5).

Day 4-5: Start incorporating breathing exercises into your daily routine (Chapter 6).

Day 6: Experiment with essential oils for snoring relief (Chapter 7).

Day 7: If you haven't found relief with the previous techniques, consider using an oral device or consult a medical professional about surgery (Chapter 8 and Chapter 9).

Remember, these changes may take time to produce results, so don't get discouraged if you don't see immediate improvements. Keep up with your efforts, and before you know it, you will be enjoying a peaceful, snore-free night's sleep.

Thank you for taking the time to read this book. I hope it has been informative and helpful in your journey toward a better night's sleep. Don't forget to

share this book with your friends and family who
may also be struggling with snoring.